Type 2 Diabetes Cookbook for the Newly Diagnosed

The Ultimate Guide to Managing Type 2 Diabetes

Dr Emily John

COPYRIGHT PAGE

TABLE OF CONTENTS

INTRODUCTION

The diagnosis of Type 2 Diabetes can be a shock to the system for anyone. Suddenly, you are forced to confront the reality that your body is not functioning the way it should, and that changes need to be made in order to manage this chronic condition. For many people, the first step in managing their Type 2 Diabetes is to take a closer look at their diet.

That's where the Type 2 Diabetes Cookbook for the Newly Diagnosed comes in. This comprehensive guide is designed specifically for those who are new to managing their Type 2 Diabetes, and are looking for practical, easy-to-follow advice on how to make the necessary dietary changes. Whether you're a seasoned cook or a complete novice in the kitchen, this book will help you develop a meal plan that works for you, and that will help you keep your blood sugar levels in check.

The first section of the book is an introduction to Type 2 Diabetes, and why diet is so important in managing this condition. We'll take a closer look at the key nutrients that are essential for people with Type 2 Diabetes, and discuss the best ways to incorporate them into your diet. We'll also cover some of the common misconceptions about Type 2 Diabetes, and explain why a low-carb, high-protein diet is often the best approach for managing this condition.

The next section of the book is all about meal planning. We'll teach you how to count carbohydrates, which is a key factor in managing blood sugar levels. You'll learn about the different types of carbohydrates, and which ones are best to include in your diet. We'll also discuss meal planning strategies, including how to plan your meals in advance, how to shop for healthy ingredients, and how to prepare healthy meals on a budget.

With the basics of meal planning covered, we'll move on to breakfast, lunch, and dinner recipes. Each recipe is designed to be easy to follow, and to incorporate the key nutrients that are essential for people with Type 2 Diabetes. You'll find a wide range of recipes to choose from, including everything from hearty breakfast casseroles to light and refreshing salads.

But we don't stop at main meals – we also include a section on snacks and desserts. Many people with Type 2 Diabetes struggle to find healthy, satisfying snacks and desserts that won't spike their blood sugar levels. Our recipes are designed to be delicious, but also to keep your blood sugar levels in check.

Of course, we understand that eating out can be a challenge for people with Type 2 Diabetes. That's why we've included a section on tips for dining out. We'll teach you how to read menus and make healthy choices, and we'll also provide some strategies for eating out with friends and family without compromising your health.

Managing your blood sugar levels is essential for people with Type 2 Diabetes, and we've included a section on strategies for doing just that. You'll learn about the different factors that can affect blood sugar levels, and we'll teach you some simple techniques for keeping your levels stable throughout the day.

Chapter 1
What is Type 2 Diabetes

Type 2 Diabetes, also known as adult-onset diabetes, is a chronic condition that affects how your body processes glucose, or blood sugar. This condition develops when the body becomes resistant to insulin or does not produce enough insulin to regulate blood sugar levels.

Insulin is a hormone produced by the pancreas that helps to regulate blood sugar levels in the body. When food is digested, glucose is released into the bloodstream. Insulin helps to move glucose from the bloodstream into the cells, where it can be used as energy or stored for later use.

When the body becomes resistant to insulin or does not produce enough insulin, glucose builds up in the bloodstream, leading to high blood sugar levels. Over time, high blood sugar levels can cause damage to organs and tissues, leading to a range of health problems.

Type 2 Diabetes is the most common type of diabetes, accounting for 90-95% of all cases of diabetes. It is most commonly diagnosed in adults over the age of 45, but can also occur in children and adolescents.

Risk factors for Type 2 Diabetes include:

- Being overweight or obese
- Having a family history of diabetes
- Being physically inactive
- Having a history of gestational diabetes (diabetes during pregnancy)
- Having polycystic ovary syndrome (PCOS)
- Having high blood pressure or high cholesterol levels
- Being of certain ethnicities, including African American, Hispanic/Latino, Native American, or Asian American

Symptoms of Type 2 Diabetes may include:

- Frequent urination

- Excessive thirst

- Fatigue

- Blurred vision

- Slow healing of wounds

- Tingling or numbness in the hands or feet

However, some people with Type 2 Diabetes may not experience any symptoms at all.

Diagnosis of Type 2 Diabetes is typically done through a blood test, which measures blood sugar levels. If blood sugar levels are higher than normal, further testing may be done to confirm a diagnosis of Type 2 Diabetes.

Treatment of Type 2 Diabetes typically involves lifestyle changes, such as diet and exercise, and medication. The goal of treatment is to regulate blood sugar levels and prevent complications associated with high blood sugar levels.

Diet plays a critical role in managing Type 2 Diabetes. A healthy diet can help regulate blood sugar levels, improve insulin sensitivity, and help manage weight. A diet for Type 2 Diabetes should be rich in whole grains, fruits, vegetables, lean protein, and healthy fats. Foods to limit include processed foods, sugary drinks, and foods high in saturated and trans fats.

Exercise is also important in managing Type 2 Diabetes. Exercise helps to improve insulin sensitivity, regulate blood sugar levels, and manage weight. The American Diabetes Association recommends at least 150 minutes of moderate-intensity aerobic exercise per week, as well as strength training exercises at least two days per week.

Medication may also be used to manage Type 2 Diabetes. Medications for Type 2 Diabetes include:

- Metformin: helps to lower blood sugar levels and improve insulin sensitivity
- Sulfonylureas: stimulate the pancreas to produce more insulin
- DPP-4 inhibitors: help to increase insulin production and decrease blood sugar levels

- GLP-1 receptor agonists: help to increase insulin production and decrease blood sugar levels
- Insulin therapy: injectable insulin may be used to regulate blood sugar levels in some cases

Complications associated with Type 2 Diabetes include:

- Heart disease and stroke: high blood sugar levels can damage blood vessels, leading to an increased risk of heart disease and stroke
- Kidney damage: high blood sugar levels can damage the kidneys, leading to kidney disease or kidney failure
- Nerve damage: high blood sugar levels can damage nerves, leading to neuropathy, or numbness and tingling in the hands and feet
- Eye damage: high blood sugar levels can damage the blood vessels in the eyes, leading to vision problems or blindness
- Foot damage: high blood sugar levels can damage the blood vessels and nerves in the feet, leading to

poor circulation and increased risk of foot infections and amputations

Prevention of Type 2 Diabetes includes maintaining a healthy weight, eating a healthy diet, and engaging in regular physical activity. Quitting smoking and managing stress levels can also help reduce the risk of developing Type 2 Diabetes.

If you have been diagnosed with Type 2 Diabetes, it is important to work closely with your healthcare team to manage your condition. Regular blood sugar monitoring, medication management, and lifestyle changes can help regulate blood sugar levels and prevent complications associated with Type 2 Diabetes.

In summary, Type 2 Diabetes is a chronic condition that affects how your body processes glucose, or blood sugar. Risk factors for Type 2 Diabetes include being overweight or obese, having a family history of diabetes, and being physically inactive. Symptoms may include frequent urination, excessive thirst, and fatigue. Treatment involves lifestyle changes, such as diet and exercise, and medication to regulate blood sugar levels. Complications associated with Type 2 Diabetes include heart disease and stroke, kidney damage, nerve damage, eye damage, and foot damage. Prevention includes maintaining a healthy weight, eating a healthy diet, and engaging in regular physical activity.

Importance of Diet in Managing Type 2 Diabetes

Diet plays a crucial role in managing type 2 diabetes. By choosing the right foods and controlling portion sizes, individuals with type 2 diabetes can regulate their blood sugar levels, improve their overall health, and reduce the risk of complications.

The key to a healthy diet for type 2 diabetes is to focus on nutrient-dense, whole foods that are rich in fiber, protein, healthy fats, vitamins, and minerals. These foods are more slowly digested and absorbed, which helps regulate blood sugar levels.

Key Nutrients to Focus on

Carbohydrates

Carbohydrates are the macronutrient that has the greatest impact on blood sugar levels. Carbohydrates are broken down into glucose, which enters the bloodstream and raises blood sugar levels.

Individuals with type 2 diabetes need to be mindful of the types and amounts of carbohydrates they consume. Complex carbohydrates, such as whole grains, fruits, vegetables, and legumes, are digested more slowly than simple carbohydrates, such as sugars and refined grains.

Fiber

Fiber is a type of carbohydrate that is not digested by the body. Instead, it passes through the digestive system, helping regulate blood sugar levels and promoting digestive health.

Foods that are high in fiber include whole grains, fruits, vegetables, legumes, nuts, and seeds. Aim to consume at least 25 grams of fiber per day.

Protein

Protein is essential for building and repairing tissues, regulating blood sugar levels, and promoting satiety. High-quality sources of protein include lean meats, poultry, fish, eggs, tofu, beans, and legumes.

Healthy Fats

Healthy fats, such as monounsaturated and polyunsaturated fats, can help regulate blood sugar levels and improve heart health. Sources of healthy fats include nuts, seeds, avocados, olive oil, and fatty fish.

Meal Planning Strategies

Meal planning is essential for individuals with type 2 diabetes to ensure they are consuming the right types and amounts of food. The following strategies can help with meal planning:

Counting Carbohydrates

Counting carbohydrates can help individuals with type 2 diabetes regulate their blood sugar levels. Carbohydrate counting involves tracking the number of carbohydrates consumed and adjusting insulin doses accordingly.

Using the Plate Method

The plate method involves dividing a plate into quarters and filling one-quarter with protein, one-quarter with whole grains, and one-half with non-starchy vegetables. This method helps ensure a balanced meal that is rich in protein, fiber, and nutrients.

Choosing Low-Glycemic Index Foods

The glycemic index is a measure of how quickly foods raise blood sugar levels. Foods with a high glycemic index, such as refined grains and sugars, should be avoided, as they cause rapid spikes in blood sugar levels. Instead, individuals with type 2 diabetes should focus on consuming foods with a low glycemic index, such as whole grains, legumes, and non-starchy vegetables.

Eating Regular Meals and Snacks

Eating regular meals and snacks can help regulate blood sugar levels and prevent overeating. Aim to consume three meals and one to two snacks per day.

Avoiding Processed Foods

Processed foods, such as packaged snacks, sugary beverages, and fast food, are often high in refined carbohydrates, sugars, and unhealthy fats. These foods should be avoided or consumed in moderation.

Planning Ahead

Planning meals and snacks ahead of time can help individuals with type 2 diabetes make healthier choices and avoid impulsive eating. Set aside time each week to plan meals and snacks, and prepare meals in advance if possible.

Chapter 2
Meal Planning

Understanding Carbohydrates

Carbohydrates are one of the three macronutrients that our bodies need to function properly, the other two being proteins and fats. Carbohydrates are composed of carbon, hydrogen, and oxygen, and they come in a variety of forms. Simple carbohydrates, such as sugar and honey, are made up of one or two sugar molecules, while complex carbohydrates, such as grains and vegetables, are made up of long chains of sugar molecules.

Carbohydrates are the primary source of energy for our bodies, and they are broken down into glucose, a type of sugar that our cells use for energy. When we consume carbohydrates, our bodies break them down into glucose, which is then transported to our cells through the bloodstream.

Different Types of Carbohydrates

Not all carbohydrates are created equal, and understanding the different types and their effects on our bodies is crucial for overall health and well-being. There are two main types of carbohydrates: simple and complex.

Simple Carbohydrates

Simple carbohydrates, also known as simple sugars, are made up of one or two sugar molecules. They are quickly digested and absorbed by our bodies, which can cause a rapid increase in blood sugar levels. Foods that are high in simple carbohydrates include sugary drinks, candy, and baked goods. While these foods can provide a quick burst of energy, they are also high in calories and can lead to weight gain and other health problems.

Complex Carbohydrates

Complex carbohydrates, also known as polysaccharides, are made up of long chains of sugar molecules. They are found in foods such as whole grains, vegetables, and legumes. Because they are more difficult for our bodies to break down and digest, complex carbohydrates provide a more sustained source of energy and help regulate blood sugar levels.

Fiber

Fiber is a type of carbohydrate that our bodies cannot digest or absorb. It is found in foods such as fruits, vegetables, whole grains, and legumes. While fiber does not provide energy like other types of carbohydrates, it is important for digestive health and can help regulate blood sugar levels. Fiber also helps us feel fuller for longer periods of time, which can aid in weight management.

The Glycemic Index

The glycemic index is a measure of how quickly a food raises blood sugar levels. Foods that are high on the glycemic index, such as white bread and sugary drinks, cause a rapid increase in blood sugar levels. Foods that are low on the glycemic index, such as whole grains and vegetables, are digested more slowly and cause a slower, more sustained increase in blood sugar levels.

The glycemic index is an important tool for people with diabetes, as it can help them make informed choices about the types of carbohydrates they consume. Foods that are high on the glycemic index should be consumed in moderation, while foods that are low on the glycemic index can be consumed more freely.

Benefits of Carbohydrates

Carbohydrates are an essential part of a healthy and balanced diet. They provide our bodies with energy, support brain function, and help regulate blood sugar levels. Carbohydrates are also a good source of fiber, which is important for digestive health and can aid in weight management.

Drawbacks of Carbohydrates

Not all carbohydrates are created equal, and some can have negative effects on our health. Foods that are high in simple carbohydrates, such as candy and sugary drinks, are high in calories and can lead to weight gain and other health problems if consumed in excess. Foods that are high on the glycemic index can also cause a rapid increase in blood sugar levels, which can be problematic for people with diabetes.

Additionally, some people may have an intolerance or sensitivity to certain types of carbohydrates, such as lactose in dairy products or gluten in wheat products. These sensitivities can cause digestive issues and other health problems.

How to Count Carbs

Carb counting involves keeping track of the amount of carbohydrates you consume each day. This can be done in a variety of ways, such as using an app or keeping a food diary. Here are the steps to follow when counting carbs:

Step 1: Determine your daily carb intake

The first step in counting carbs is to determine how many carbs you should be consuming each day. This will vary depending on factors such as age, sex, weight, height, and activity level. Your healthcare provider can help you determine your daily carb intake. In general, the American Diabetes Association recommends that people with Type 2

Diabetes consume between 45-60 grams of carbs per meal, or 135-180 grams of carbs per day.

Step 2: Learn how to read food labels

The next step is to learn how to read food labels. Food labels provide information about the amount of carbohydrates in a particular food item. Look for the "Total Carbohydrates" section on the label. This will tell you how many grams of carbohydrates are in one serving of the food.

Step 3: Measure your food

To accurately count carbs, you need to know how much food you're consuming. This can be done by measuring your food using a food scale or measuring cups. For example, if you're eating pasta, measure out one serving size using a measuring cup.

Step 4: Add up your carbs

Once you know how many carbs are in one serving of a particular food item and how much you're consuming, you can add up your carbs. For example, if one serving of pasta has 30 grams of carbs and you're eating two servings, you'll consume 60 grams of carbs.

Step 5: Adjust your insulin or medication dosage

After you've counted your carbs, you may need to adjust your insulin or medication dosage. Your healthcare provider can help you determine how much insulin or medication you need based on your carb intake. This will help you manage your blood sugar levels and prevent spikes.

Tips for Getting Started with Carb Counting

If you're new to carb counting, it can be overwhelming at first. Here are some tips to help you get started:

- Keep a food diary: Write down everything you eat and the number of carbs in each item. This will help you track your carb intake and identify any patterns or trends.
- Use a carb counting app: There are many carb counting apps available that can help you track your carb intake. These apps can also provide nutritional

information about food items and help you make healthier choices.

- Be consistent: Try to eat meals and snacks at the same time every day. This can help you better manage your blood sugar levels and make it easier to track your carb intake.

- Avoid processed foods: Processed foods often contain high amounts of sugar and carbs. Instead, opt for whole, unprocessed foods like fruits, vegetables, and whole grains.

- Seek support: Managing Type 2 Diabetes can be challenging. Don't be afraid to seek support from family, friends, or a healthcare provider. They can provide you with the guidance and encouragement you need to succeed.

Meal Planning Strategies

Meal planning is an essential component of managing Type 2 diabetes. Whether you have recently been diagnosed or have been living with diabetes for years, planning your meals can help you maintain healthy blood sugar levels and manage your weight. In this article, we will explore some effective meal planning strategies that can help you maintain your blood sugar levels, eat healthily, and feel satisfied.

Start with a Plan: One of the most important meal planning strategies is to start with a plan. Create a meal plan for the week that includes breakfast, lunch, dinner, and snacks. Write down the meals you plan to eat, and be sure to include the ingredients you will need. This will help you stay organized and ensure that you have all the necessary ingredients on hand.

When planning your meals, consider your schedule for the week. For example, if you have a busy week ahead, plan for meals that can be prepared quickly or cooked in advance. You may also want to plan for leftovers that can be reheated for a quick and easy meal.

Focus on Nutrient-Dense Foods: When planning your meals, focus on nutrient-dense foods. These are foods that are high in vitamins, minerals, and other essential nutrients but are low in calories. Nutrient-dense foods include vegetables, fruits, whole grains, lean proteins, and healthy fats.

Vegetables should be the foundation of your meals, as they are low in calories, high in fiber, and packed with nutrients. Aim for a variety of colorful vegetables, such as leafy greens, broccoli, peppers, carrots, and sweet potatoes. Fruits are also a great source of nutrients, but be mindful of their sugar content. Stick to low-sugar fruits, such as berries, apples, and citrus fruits.

Whole grains are another important source of nutrients, as they are high in fiber, vitamins, and minerals. Opt for whole-grain bread, pasta, and rice, and choose cereals that are low in sugar and high in fiber. Lean proteins, such as chicken, fish, and tofu, are important for maintaining muscle mass and providing essential amino acids. Healthy fats, such as olive oil, avocado, and nuts, are important for brain function and overall health.

Balance Your Meals: Balancing your meals is another important meal planning strategy. Aim for a combination of carbohydrates, protein, and healthy fats at each meal. Carbohydrates are important for providing energy, but be mindful of their impact on blood sugar levels. Choose complex carbohydrates, such as whole grains and vegetables, over refined carbohydrates, such as white bread and sugar.

Protein is important for maintaining muscle mass and providing essential amino acids. Aim for lean sources of protein, such as chicken, fish, and tofu. Healthy fats are important for brain function and overall health. Choose sources of healthy fats, such as olive oil, avocado, and nuts.

Plan for Snacks: Snacks are an important part of meal planning, as they can help you maintain your blood sugar levels and prevent overeating at meals. Plan for snacks that are high in protein and fiber, such as a piece of fruit with a handful of nuts or a hard-boiled egg with vegetables. Avoid snacks that are high in sugar, such as candy and soda.

Meal Prep: Meal prep is another important meal planning strategy. Set aside time each week to prepare meals in advance. This can include chopping vegetables, cooking rice and quinoa, and marinating chicken. By preparing meals in advance, you can save time during the week and ensure that you have healthy meals on hand.

Mindful Eating: Finally, mindful eating is an important component of meal planning. Mindful eating means being present and aware of your food, your body, and your surroundings. It means taking the time to savor your food, paying attention to its flavors, textures, and smells. Mindful eating also means paying attention to your hunger and fullness cues, eating slowly, and stopping when you feel full.

To practice mindful eating, try to eat without distractions, such as watching TV or working on your computer. Instead, sit down at a table and focus on your food. Take small bites, chew slowly, and put your utensils down between bites. This will help you eat more slowly, which can help you feel more satisfied and prevent overeating.

Chapter 3

Breakfast

Breakfast is considered the most important meal of the day as it fuels your body for the day ahead. Eating breakfast can help you stay energized, focused, and productive throughout the day. For those who have recently been diagnosed with type 2 diabetes, choosing the right breakfast can be challenging. However, there are plenty of delicious breakfast recipes that are both nutritious and easy to make. In this article, we will explore some of the best breakfast recipes for those who are newly diagnosed with type 2 diabetes.

Avocado Toast: Avocado toast is a popular breakfast dish that is both tasty and nutritious. To make avocado toast, you will need:

Ingredients:

- 1 slice of whole-grain bread

- 1 ripe avocado

- 1 tsp. of olive oil

- Salt and pepper to taste

Instructions:

1. Toast the bread until it is golden brown.

2. Cut the avocado in half, remove the pit, and scoop out the flesh into a bowl.

3. Mash the avocado with a fork until it is smooth.

4. Add the olive oil, salt, and pepper to the mashed avocado and mix well.

5. Spread the avocado mixture on the toasted bread and serve.

Avocado is rich in healthy fats, fiber, and vitamins, making it an excellent choice for a healthy breakfast.

Greek Yogurt with Berries: Greek yogurt with berries is another delicious and healthy breakfast recipe that is perfect for those with type 2 diabetes. To make Greek yogurt with berries, you will need:

Ingredients:

- 1 cup of plain Greek yogurt
- 1/2 cup of mixed berries (strawberries, blueberries, raspberries, etc.)
- 1 tbsp. of honey
- 1/4 cup of granola

Instructions:

1. Place the Greek yogurt in a bowl.
2. Wash and chop the berries and add them to the bowl with the yogurt.
3. Drizzle the honey over the top of the yogurt and berries.
4. Sprinkle the granola over the top of the yogurt and berries and serve.

Greek yogurt is high in protein, calcium, and probiotics, making it an excellent choice for a healthy breakfast. Berries are also high in fiber and antioxidants, making them a great addition to this recipe.

Omelet with Vegetables: Omelets are a popular breakfast dish that can be customized with a variety of vegetables to make them more nutritious. To make an omelet with vegetables, you will need:

Ingredients:

- 2 eggs
- 1/4 cup of chopped vegetables (spinach, onions, peppers, mushrooms, etc.)
- 1 tsp. of olive oil
- Salt and pepper to taste

Instructions:

1. Heat the olive oil in a small skillet over medium heat.
2. Add the chopped vegetables to the skillet and sauté for 2-3 minutes until they are tender.
3. In a small bowl, whisk together the eggs and add them to the skillet with the vegetables.

4. Cook the eggs for 2-3 minutes until they start to set.

5. Use a spatula to fold the omelet in half and continue cooking for another minute until the eggs are fully cooked.

6. Season the omelet with salt and pepper and serve.

Vegetables are a great source of fiber, vitamins, and minerals, making this omelet a healthy breakfast option for those with type 2 diabetes.

Overnight Oats: Overnight oats are a quick and easy breakfast recipe that can be prepared the night before and enjoyed in the morning. To make overnight oats, you will need:

Ingredients:

- 1/2 cup of rolled oats
- 1/2 cup of almond milk
- 1/2 cup of plain Greek yogurt
- 1/2 cup of mixed berries
- 1 tbsp. of chia seeds

- 1 tbsp. of honey

- 1/4 tsp. of cinnamon

Instructions:

1. In a mason jar or bowl, combine the rolled oats, almond milk, Greek yogurt, chia seeds, honey, and cinnamon.
2. Stir the ingredients together until well combined.
3. Add the mixed berries to the jar or bowl and stir gently.
4. Cover the jar or bowl with a lid or plastic wrap and refrigerate overnight.
5. In the morning, stir the ingredients together again and enjoy.

This recipe is high in fiber, protein, and healthy fats, making it a great breakfast option for those with type 2 diabetes.

Sweet Potato Hash: Sweet potato hash is a savory breakfast dish that is both delicious and nutritious. To make sweet potato hash, you will need:

Ingredients:

- 1 medium sweet potato, peeled and diced
- 1/4 cup of diced onion
- 1/4 cup of diced bell pepper
- 2 slices of turkey bacon, diced
- 1 tsp. of olive oil
- Salt and pepper to taste

Instructions:

1. Heat the olive oil in a skillet over medium heat.
2. Add the diced sweet potato to the skillet and sauté for 8-10 minutes until it is tender and slightly browned.
3. Add the diced onion, bell pepper, and turkey bacon to the skillet and sauté for an additional 3-5 minutes

until the vegetables are tender and the bacon is crispy.

4. Season the sweet potato hash with salt and pepper and serve.

Sweet potatoes are a great source of fiber, vitamins, and minerals, making them a healthy breakfast option for those with type 2 diabetes.

Choosing the right breakfast can be challenging for those who have recently been diagnosed with type 2 diabetes. However, there are plenty of delicious and healthy breakfast recipes that can be enjoyed by those with this condition. From avocado toast to sweet potato hash, there are plenty of options to choose from that are high in fiber, protein, and healthy fats. By incorporating these recipes into your breakfast routine, you can start your day off right and maintain good health.

Tips for Making Breakfast Healthier

A healthy breakfast can help to set the tone for the rest of your day, providing you with the energy and nutrients needed to perform at your best. However, not all breakfasts are created equal, and it's easy to fall into the trap of choosing high-sugar, high-fat, and high-calorie options. If you're looking to make your breakfasts healthier, then you've come to the right place. we'll explore some tips and tricks to help you make your breakfasts more nutritious and satisfying.

Tip 1: Choose Whole Grains

One of the easiest ways to make your breakfast healthier is to choose whole grains. Whole grains are a great source of fiber, vitamins, and minerals and can help to keep you feeling full and satisfied throughout the morning. Examples of whole grain breakfast options include:

- Whole grain toast or English muffins
- Oatmeal or steel-cut oats
- Whole grain pancakes or waffles
- Brown rice or quinoa bowls
- Whole grain cereal with milk or yogurt

When shopping for whole grain products, be sure to check the label and choose items that are made with 100% whole grains. Some products may be labeled as "multigrain" or "wheat," but unless they specifically say "whole grain," they may not be as healthy as you think.

Tip 2: Incorporate Protein

Protein is an essential nutrient that helps to build and repair tissues in the body. It can also help to keep you feeling full and satisfied throughout the morning, preventing overeating and snacking on unhealthy options. Some protein-rich breakfast options include:

- Eggs (scrambled, boiled, or omelet)
- Greek yogurt or cottage cheese
- Nut butter on toast or whole grain waffles
- Protein smoothie with protein powder, fruit, and milk or yogurt
- Tofu or tempeh scramble with vegetables

If you're not a fan of traditional protein sources, there are plenty of plant-based options available, such as nuts, seeds, and beans.

Tip 3: Add Colorful Fruits and Vegetables

Fruits and vegetables are packed with vitamins, minerals, and antioxidants, making them an essential part of any healthy breakfast. They can also add flavor, texture, and color to your meal. Some colorful fruit and vegetable breakfast options include:

- Smoothie bowls with fruit, yogurt, and greens
- Avocado toast with tomato and basil
- Fresh fruit salad with yogurt or cottage cheese
- Omelets or scrambles with vegetables like spinach, mushrooms, and bell peppers
- Breakfast burrito with black beans, salsa, and avocado

When choosing fruits and vegetables, try to choose a variety of colors to ensure that you're getting a wide range of nutrients.

Tip 4: Cut Back on Sugar

Many traditional breakfast options, such as pastries, cereals, and granola bars, are loaded with sugar. While sugar can provide a quick burst of energy, it can also lead to a crash and leave you feeling hungry and sluggish. To cut back on sugar, try:

- Choosing plain or low-sugar cereals or oatmeal
- Skipping the flavored creamers in your coffee and opting for milk or a natural sweetener like honey or maple syrup
- Avoiding sugary pastries and baked goods and opting for whole grain toast or a protein-rich option instead
- Making your own granola or energy bars with natural sweeteners like dates or bananas

While it's okay to indulge in sugary treats occasionally, making them a regular part of your breakfast routine can sabotage your health goals.

Tip 5: Experiment with Spices and Herbs

Adding spices and herbs to your breakfast can add flavor and nutrition without adding calories or fat. Spices and herbs like cinnamon, nutmeg, turmeric, and ginger are known for their anti-inflammatory and antioxidant properties. Some ideas for using spices and herbs in your breakfast include:

- Sprinkling cinnamon on oatmeal or yogurt
- Adding turmeric and ginger to smoothies or oatmeal
- Using fresh herbs like basil or cilantro in omelets or scrambles
- Adding a dash of nutmeg to pancakes or waffles

Not only do spices and herbs add flavor and nutrition to your breakfast, but they can also help to reduce inflammation and support overall health.

Tip 6: Prep Your Breakfast Ahead of Time

One of the biggest challenges to eating a healthy breakfast is time. With busy schedules and rushed mornings, it's easy to grab something quick and unhealthy. However, taking the time to prep your breakfast ahead of time can make all the difference. Some ideas for prepping your breakfast ahead of time include:

- Making overnight oats or chia seed pudding
- Preparing breakfast burritos or sandwiches and freezing them for quick reheating
- Baking a batch of muffins or breakfast bars on the weekend and grabbing one on busy mornings
- Chopping vegetables and prepping ingredients for smoothies the night before

By prepping your breakfast ahead of time, you can ensure that you have a healthy and satisfying option ready to go, even on the busiest of mornings.

Tip 7: Don't Skip Breakfast

Perhaps the most important tip for making your breakfast healthier is simply not to skip it altogether. Skipping breakfast can lead to overeating later in the day, as well as poor concentration, low energy, and a slowed metabolism. Even if you don't have time for a sit-down meal, try to grab something quick and healthy on the go, such as a piece of fruit, a protein bar, or a smoothie.

Lunch Recipes

Lunch is an essential meal that gives us the energy and nutrients we need to power through the rest of the day. When you are dealing with a condition like Type 2 Diabetes, it is even more important to make sure your lunch is healthy and balanced.

In this chapter, we will explore a range of delicious and nutritious lunch recipes that are perfect for anyone who has recently been diagnosed with Type 2 Diabetes. We will provide a detailed breakdown of the ingredients and the nutritional value of each recipe, as well as tips on how to prepare and serve them.

Grilled Chicken Salad: Grilled chicken salad is a classic lunch recipe that is both filling and healthy. To make this dish, you will need:

Ingredients:

- 2 boneless, skinless chicken breasts
- 1 tbsp. olive oil
- Salt and pepper to taste
- 4 cups mixed greens
- 1 cup cherry tomatoes, halved
- 1 avocado, sliced
- 2 tbsp. balsamic vinegar
- 1 tbsp. Dijon mustard

Instructions:

1. Preheat a grill or grill pan to medium-high heat.
2. Brush the chicken breasts with olive oil and season with salt and pepper.
3. Grill the chicken for 6-8 minutes per side, or until cooked through.
4. Let the chicken cool for a few minutes before slicing it into strips.
5. In a large bowl, combine the mixed greens, cherry tomatoes, and avocado slices.

6. In a small bowl, whisk together the balsamic vinegar and Dijon mustard.

7. Drizzle the dressing over the salad and toss to combine.

8. Add the sliced chicken on top of the salad and serve.

This grilled chicken salad is high in protein and healthy fats, making it a great choice for anyone who is looking to manage their blood sugar levels. The balsamic vinegar and Dijon mustard dressing is a delicious and low-sugar alternative to traditional dressings that are high in added sugars.

Turkey and Hummus Wrap: Wraps are a great option for a healthy and portable lunch that can be eaten on-the-go. This turkey and hummus wrap is packed with protein and healthy fats, and can be made in just a few minutes. To make this recipe, you will need:

Ingredients:

- 1 large whole wheat tortilla
- 3 oz. sliced turkey breast
- 1/4 cup hummus
- 1/4 cup shredded carrots
- 1/4 cup sliced cucumber
- 1/4 cup baby spinach leaves
- Salt and pepper to taste

Instructions:

1. Lay the whole wheat tortilla flat on a plate.
2. Spread the hummus evenly over the tortilla, leaving a 1-inch border around the edge.
3. Layer the sliced turkey breast, shredded carrots, sliced cucumber, and baby spinach leaves on top of the hummus.
4. Season with salt and pepper to taste.
5. Roll the tortilla up tightly, tucking in the edges as you go.
6. Slice the wrap in half and serve.

This turkey and hummus wrap is a great alternative to traditional deli sandwiches that are often high in added sugars and unhealthy fats. The hummus provides a healthy source of protein and fiber, while the shredded carrots and sliced cucumber add a delicious crunch.

Tuna Salad Lettuce Wraps: If you are looking for a low-carb and high-protein lunch option, these tuna salad lettuce wraps are a great choice. To make this recipe, you will need:

Ingredients:

- 2 cans of tuna, drained
- 1/4 cup mayonnaise
- 1/4 cup diced celery
- 2 tbsp. diced red onion
- 1 tbsp. Dijon mustard
- 1 tsp. lemon juice
- Salt and pepper to taste
- Butter lettuce leaves

Instructions:

1. In a medium-sized bowl, combine the drained tuna, mayonnaise, diced celery, diced red onion, Dijon mustard, lemon juice, salt, and pepper.
2. Stir the ingredients together until they are well combined.
3. Take a butter lettuce leaf and spoon the tuna salad onto it, spreading it out evenly.
4. Roll the lettuce leaf up tightly, tucking in the sides as you go.
5. Repeat with the remaining lettuce leaves and tuna salad.
6. Serve chilled.

These tuna salad lettuce wraps are a great option for anyone who is looking for a low-carb and high-protein lunch. The tuna provides a healthy source of omega-3 fatty acids, while the celery and red onion add a delicious crunch. The Dijon mustard and lemon juice give the tuna salad a tangy flavor that is both delicious and refreshing.

Vegetarian Quinoa Bowl: For anyone who is looking for a vegetarian lunch option that is packed with protein, this quinoa bowl is a great choice. To make this recipe, you will need:

Ingredients:

- 1 cup quinoa
- 1 can black beans, drained and rinsed
- 1 red bell pepper, diced
- 1 yellow bell pepper, diced
- 1 avocado, diced
- 1/4 cup chopped cilantro
- 2 tbsp. olive oil
- 1 tbsp. lime juice
- Salt and pepper to taste

Instructions:

1. Cook the quinoa according to the instructions on the package.

2. In a large bowl, combine the cooked quinoa, black beans, diced red and yellow bell peppers, and diced avocado.

3. In a small bowl, whisk together the olive oil, lime juice, salt, and pepper.

4. Pour the dressing over the quinoa mixture and toss to combine.

5. Sprinkle the chopped cilantro on top of the quinoa bowl and serve.

This vegetarian quinoa bowl is a great choice for anyone who is looking to increase their intake of plant-based proteins. The quinoa and black beans provide a healthy source of protein and fiber, while the bell peppers and avocado add a delicious crunch. The lime juice and cilantro give the dish a zesty flavor that is both refreshing and satisfying.

Lunch is an important meal that can have a significant impact on our overall health and well-being. When you are dealing with a condition like Type 2 Diabetes, it is especially important to make sure that your lunch is healthy and balanced.

The recipes we have provided in this chapter are all delicious and nutritious, and are perfect for anyone who has recently been diagnosed with Type 2 Diabetes. Whether you are looking for a high-protein salad, a low-carb wrap, or a vegetarian quinoa bowl, we have got you covered.

By making small changes to your lunchtime routine, you can take control of your health and manage your blood sugar levels more effectively. So why not try out one of these delicious lunch recipes today and see how easy it can be to eat healthy and stay on track with your health goals.

Tips for Packing a Healthy Lunch

Many people find it challenging to pack a healthy lunch, especially if they are in a rush or don't have access to a kitchen. In this article, we will provide you with some tips for packing a healthy lunch that is easy, delicious, and nutritious.

Plan Ahead

The first step in packing a healthy lunch is to plan ahead. You should set aside some time each week to plan out your meals and snacks. This will help you avoid making poor food choices when you are hungry and in a rush. When planning your meals, think about what foods will provide you with the most energy and nutrients. Try to include a variety of foods from different food groups, such as fruits, vegetables, whole grains, and lean protein.

Choose the Right Container

Choosing the right container for your lunch is essential. You want a container that is sturdy, leak-proof, and easy to transport. Consider investing in a reusable lunch container that has separate compartments for different foods. This will help you avoid mixing your foods and keep them fresh until lunchtime. You can also use insulated containers to keep your food hot or cold, depending on your preference.

Include a Variety of Foods

To ensure that you are getting all the nutrients you need, it's important to include a variety of foods in your lunch. You should aim to include at least one serving of fruits and vegetables in each meal. Try to choose colorful fruits and vegetables, as they are often rich in nutrients. You can also include whole grains, such as brown rice or quinoa, as well as lean protein, such as chicken or fish.

Pack Healthy Snacks

In addition to your main meal, you should also pack healthy snacks to munch on throughout the day. Snacks can help you maintain your energy levels and prevent you from overeating during your next meal. Choose healthy snacks that are high in protein and fiber, such as nuts, seeds, or fruit. You can also pack some cut-up vegetables and hummus, which is a tasty and healthy snack.

Avoid Processed Foods

Processed foods, such as chips and cookies, are often high in sugar, salt, and unhealthy fats. They can also be low in nutrients, which can lead to weight gain and other health problems. Instead of processed foods, try to pack whole foods that are fresh and unprocessed. This will ensure that you are getting all the nutrients you need to stay healthy and energized.

Don't Forget to Hydrate

Drinking enough water throughout the day is essential for maintaining your energy levels and preventing dehydration. You should aim to drink at least eight glasses of water per day. You can also include some herbal tea or coconut water in your lunch to help you stay hydrated.

Get Creative with Your Meals

Packing a healthy lunch doesn't have to be boring. You can get creative with your meals and try new recipes. Look for healthy lunch recipes online or in cookbooks, and experiment with different flavors and ingredients. You can also try making your own salad dressings or dips, which are often healthier and more delicious than store-bought versions.

Dinner Recipes

Dinner is an essential meal of the day, as it is typically the last meal that people have before going to bed. Therefore, it is crucial to have a nutritious and healthy dinner to maintain a balanced diet. A well-planned dinner should provide the necessary nutrients to the body and should be easy to digest. In this article, we will provide some unique and delicious dinner recipes that are healthy and easy to prepare.

Recipe 1: Grilled Salmon with Asparagus and Quinoa

Ingredients:

- 4 salmon fillets (6 oz each)
- 1 lb asparagus
- 1 cup quinoa
- 2 cups water

- 1 tsp salt

- 1 tsp black pepper

- 2 tbsp olive oil

- 1 tbsp lemon juice

- 1 tbsp honey

- 2 garlic cloves, minced

Instructions:

1. Preheat the grill to medium-high heat.

2. Rinse the quinoa and add it to a saucepan with 2 cups of water and 1 tsp salt. Bring to a boil and reduce the heat to low, cover the pan and let it simmer for 15-20 minutes, or until the water is absorbed.

3. Rinse the salmon fillets and pat dry with a paper towel. Season with salt and pepper.

4. Snap the ends of the asparagus and drizzle with olive oil.

5. In a small bowl, whisk together the lemon juice, honey, garlic, and olive oil.

6. Grill the salmon for 5-6 minutes on each side or until the salmon is cooked through.

7. Grill the asparagus for 5-6 minutes or until they are tender.

8. Fluff the quinoa with a fork and add it to a serving dish.

9. Arrange the grilled salmon and asparagus on top of the quinoa and drizzle the lemon-honey-garlic sauce over it.

Recipe 2: Mediterranean Chicken Skewers with Tzatziki Sauce

Ingredients:

- 1 lb boneless, skinless chicken breast
- 1 red bell pepper
- 1 yellow bell pepper
- 1 onion
- 1 tbsp olive oil
- 1 tsp dried oregano
- 1 tsp dried thyme

- 1 tsp garlic powder

- 1 tsp salt

- 1/2 tsp black pepper

- Wooden skewers

- For the tzatziki sauce:

- 1/2 cup Greek yogurt

- 1/2 cup diced cucumber

- 1 garlic clove, minced

- 1 tbsp chopped fresh dill

- 1 tbsp lemon juice

- Salt and black pepper to taste

Instructions:

1. Cut the chicken breast into 1-inch cubes.

2. Cut the bell peppers and onion into bite-size pieces.

3. In a bowl, whisk together the olive oil, oregano, thyme, garlic powder, salt, and black pepper.

4. Add the chicken and vegetables to the bowl and mix well to coat them with the marinade.

5. Cover the bowl with plastic wrap and let it marinate in the refrigerator for at least 30 minutes.

6. Preheat the grill to medium-high heat.

7. Thread the chicken and vegetables onto wooden skewers.

8. Grill the skewers for 8-10 minutes or until the chicken is cooked through.

9. To make the tzatziki sauce, mix together the Greek yogurt, cucumber, garlic, dill, lemon juice, salt, and black pepper.

10. Serve the skewers with the tzatziki sauce on the side.

Recipe 3: Vegetarian Stuffed Peppers

Ingredients:

- 4 bell peppers
- 1 cup quinoa
- 2 cups water
- 1/2 onion, diced
- 2 garlic cloves, minced
- 1 zucchini, diced
- 1 carrot, diced

- 1/2 cup frozen corn

- 1/2 cup black beans, drained and rinsed

- 1/2 cup diced tomatoes

- 1 tsp ground cumin

- 1 tsp paprika

- Salt and black pepper to taste

- 1/4 cup shredded cheddar cheese (optional)

Instructions:

1. Preheat the oven to 375°F.
2. Cut the top off the bell peppers and remove the seeds and membranes.
3. Rinse the quinoa and add it to a saucepan with 2 cups of water. Bring to a boil and reduce the heat to low, cover the pan and let it simmer for 15-20 minutes, or until the water is absorbed.
4. In a skillet, heat olive oil over medium heat. Add the onion and garlic and sauté for 2-3 minutes.
5. Add the zucchini, carrot, corn, black beans, diced tomatoes, ground cumin, paprika, salt, and black

pepper. Cook for 5-7 minutes or until the vegetables are tender.

6. Add the cooked quinoa to the skillet and stir to combine.

7. Stuff the bell peppers with the quinoa-vegetable mixture and place them in a baking dish.

8. Cover the dish with foil and bake for 30-40 minutes or until the peppers are tender.

9. If desired, sprinkle shredded cheddar cheese on top of the peppers and bake for an additional 5 minutes or until the cheese is melted and bubbly.

Dinner is an important meal of the day, and it is essential to make it nutritious and healthy. These dinner recipes are easy to prepare and full of essential nutrients that are necessary for a balanced diet. Whether you are a meat lover or a vegetarian, there is a recipe for everyone to enjoy. So, try these recipes and make your dinner healthy and delicious!

Tips for Making Healthy Dinner Choices

In this chapter, we will share some valuable tips for making healthy dinner choices. With these tips, you can create healthy and nutritious meals that are easy to prepare, delicious, and perfect for you and your family.

1. Include a Variety of Colors in Your Meals

Incorporating a variety of colors in your meals is an excellent way to make healthy dinner choices. Fruits and vegetables of different colors contain different nutrients, vitamins, and minerals. By including a variety of colors in your meals, you can ensure that your body receives all the nutrients it needs.

When planning your meals, aim to incorporate different colored fruits and vegetables such as red peppers, green spinach, yellow squash, and purple cabbage. Mix and match different colors to create visually appealing meals that are nutritious and delicious.

2.   Use Whole Foods

One of the best ways to make healthy dinner choices is to use whole foods. Whole foods are foods that are minimally processed and do not contain added sugars or chemicals. Examples of whole foods include fruits, vegetables, whole grains, and lean proteins. These foods provide your body with essential nutrients, vitamins, and minerals.

When grocery shopping, choose fresh fruits and vegetables, whole grains such as brown rice, whole-grain bread, and pasta. Opt for lean proteins such as chicken, turkey, fish, and beans. Avoid processed meats, such as bacon and sausages, as they contain high levels of salt and saturated fats.

3.   Choose Healthy Fats

Fats are an essential part of a healthy diet. However, it is essential to choose healthy fats over unhealthy fats. Healthy fats such as monounsaturated and polyunsaturated fats provide our bodies with essential nutrients, support heart health, and help reduce inflammation. Examples of foods that contain healthy fats include avocados, nuts, seeds, olive oil, and fatty fish such as salmon.

Avoid unhealthy fats such as saturated fats and trans fats. These fats increase cholesterol levels and increase the risk of heart disease. Examples of foods that contain unhealthy fats include fried foods, processed foods, and baked goods.

4.   Limit Processed Foods

Processed foods are foods that have undergone significant processing, typically to increase their shelf life. Processed foods often contain high levels of sodium, sugar, and unhealthy fats, which can lead to weight gain, heart disease, and other chronic illnesses.

When making healthy dinner choices, limit processed foods as much as possible. Instead, opt for fresh and minimally processed foods. If you must consume processed foods, check the labels carefully, and choose foods with lower levels of salt, sugar, and unhealthy fats.

5.   Watch Your Portion Sizes

Portion sizes play a significant role in making healthy dinner choices. Consuming large portions of food can lead to overeating and weight gain. It is essential to watch your portion sizes and consume the right amount of food for your body's needs.

When preparing your meals, aim to fill half your plate with fruits and vegetables, a quarter with lean protein, and a quarter with whole grains or starchy vegetables such as sweet potatoes. Avoid overeating by using smaller plates, measuring your food, and avoiding distractions such as the television or phone while eating.

6.   Experiment with Different Cooking Techniques

Experimenting with different cooking techniques is an excellent way to make healthy dinner choices. Cooking techniques such as grilling, broiling, and roasting can help retain the nutrients in your food and reduce the need for added fats and oils.

Try grilling your chicken or fish instead of frying it. Roast your vegetables in the oven with a drizzle of olive oil and herbs instead of boiling them. Experiment with different seasoning blends to add flavor to your meals without adding extra salt or sugar.

making healthy dinner choices is essential for maintaining good health and reducing the risk of chronic illnesses. By planning your meals ahead of time, using whole foods, choosing healthy fats, limiting processed foods, watching your portion sizes, experimenting with different cooking techniques, including

Chapter 6

Snacks and Desserts

Snack Ideas and Recipes

Snacking is an essential part of our daily routine. For some, it's a way to satisfy hunger pangs between meals, while for others, it's an enjoyable way to break the monotony of a long workday. However, for people with Type 2 Diabetes, snacking can be a challenging task. Most of the store-bought snacks are packed with unhealthy ingredients such as refined sugar, trans-fat, and artificial flavors. These ingredients can spike up the blood sugar levels and make it difficult to manage diabetes.

But don't worry! There are plenty of healthy and tasty snack options available that are perfect for people with Type 2 Diabetes. In this chapter, we will explore some of the best snack ideas and recipes that are easy to make, delicious, and most importantly, diabetes-friendly.

Greek Yogurt with Berries: Greek yogurt is an excellent source of protein and calcium, which makes it an ideal snack option for people with diabetes. When paired with berries, it provides a healthy dose of fiber and antioxidants, which help to regulate blood sugar levels and boost immunity.

Ingredients:

- 1 cup of plain Greek yogurt
- 1/2 cup of mixed berries (strawberries, blueberries, and raspberries)
- 1 tablespoon of honey (optional)

Instructions:

1. In a small bowl, mix the Greek yogurt and honey until well combined.
2. Top it with mixed berries.
3. Enjoy!

Apple Slices with Almond Butter: Apple slices with almond butter are a perfect combination of sweet and salty flavors. Almond butter is rich in healthy fats, fiber, and protein, which helps to slow down the digestion process and prevent blood sugar spikes.

Ingredients:

- 1 medium-sized apple
- 2 tablespoons of almond butter
- A pinch of cinnamon powder (optional)

Instructions:

1. Cut the apple into thin slices.
2. Spread almond butter on each slice.
3. Sprinkle a pinch of cinnamon powder (optional)
4. Enjoy!

Roasted Chickpeas: Roasted chickpeas are a healthy and crunchy snack that is rich in protein and fiber. They are easy to make and can be seasoned with your favorite spices to add a unique flavor.

Ingredients:

- 1 can of chickpeas (15 oz)
- 1 tablespoon of olive oil
- 1/2 teaspoon of cumin powder
- 1/2 teaspoon of paprika powder
- Salt and pepper to taste

Instructions:

1. Preheat the oven to 400°F.
2. Rinse the chickpeas and pat them dry with a paper towel.
3. In a bowl, mix the chickpeas, olive oil, cumin powder, paprika powder, salt, and pepper.
4. Spread the chickpeas in a single layer on a baking sheet.
5. Roast them for 25-30 minutes until crispy.
6. Enjoy!

Hummus with Veggies: Hummus is a creamy and delicious dip that is made from chickpeas, tahini, lemon juice, and olive oil. It is rich in protein, fiber, and healthy fats, which makes it a perfect snack option for people with diabetes. When paired with veggies, it provides a healthy dose of vitamins and minerals, which helps to improve overall health.

Ingredients:

- 1 can of chickpeas (15 oz)
- 1/4 cup of tahini
- 2 cloves of garlic
- 2 tablespoons of lemon juice
- 2 tablespoons of olive oil
- Salt and pepper to taste
- Carrots, cucumbers, and celery sticks for dipping

Instructions:

1. Rinse the chickpeas and pat them dry with a paper towel.

2. In a food processor, blend the chickpeas, tahini, garlic, lemon juice, olive oil, salt, and pepper until smooth and creamy.

3. If the mixture is too thick, add a tablespoon of water at a time until it reaches your desired consistency.

4. Transfer the hummus to a bowl and serve with carrot sticks, cucumber slices, and celery sticks for dipping.

5. Enjoy!

Turkey Roll-Ups: Turkey roll-ups are a tasty and low-carb snack that is easy to make and perfect for people with diabetes. They are a good source of protein and healthy fats, which helps to keep you feeling full for longer.

Ingredients:

- 4 slices of turkey breast
- 2 tablespoons of cream cheese
- 1/2 teaspoon of dried basil
- 1/2 teaspoon of dried oregano
- Salt and pepper to taste

- Spinach leaves

Instructions:

1. In a small bowl, mix the cream cheese, dried basil, dried oregano, salt, and pepper until well combined.
2. Lay the turkey slices on a cutting board.
3. Spread the cream cheese mixture on each slice.
4. Top with spinach leaves.
5. Roll up tightly and secure with a toothpick.
6. Enjoy!

Hard-Boiled Eggs: Hard-boiled eggs are a simple and protein-packed snack that is perfect for people with diabetes. They are easy to make and can be stored in the fridge for up to a week, making them a convenient snack option for on-the-go.

Ingredients:

- 2 large eggs
- Salt and pepper to taste

Instructions:

1. Place the eggs in a saucepan and cover them with water.
2. Bring the water to a boil over high heat.
3. Reduce the heat to low and simmer for 10 minutes.
4. Drain the water and run the eggs under cold water to cool them down.
5. Peel the eggs and sprinkle with salt and pepper.
6. Enjoy!

Cottage Cheese with Pineapple: Cottage cheese with pineapple is a sweet and creamy snack that is rich in protein and calcium. Pineapple contains an enzyme called bromelain, which helps to aid digestion and reduce inflammation.

Ingredients:

- 1/2 cup of low-fat cottage cheese
- 1/2 cup of fresh pineapple chunks

Instructions:

1. In a small bowl, mix the cottage cheese and pineapple chunks.
2. Enjoy!

Snacking can be a healthy and enjoyable experience for people with diabetes. By choosing snacks that are high in protein, fiber, and healthy fats, you can regulate blood sugar levels and improve overall health. Try out these snack ideas and recipes to add some variety to your snacking routine and satisfy your cravings without compromising your health.

Dessert Ideas and Recipes

Desserts are the perfect way to end a meal, and they don't have to be unhealthy. With a little creativity and the right ingredients, you can indulge in your sweet tooth without sabotaging your diet. Here are some delicious dessert ideas and recipes that are perfect for those with a sweet tooth.

Chocolate Avocado Pudding

This rich and creamy chocolate pudding is made with avocados and sweetened with honey, making it a healthy and satisfying dessert option. To make the pudding, simply blend together avocados, cocoa powder, honey, vanilla extract, and almond milk until smooth. Chill the pudding in the refrigerator for at least an hour before serving. For an extra treat, top with fresh berries or sliced almonds.

Strawberry Shortcake

This classic dessert is a crowd-pleaser, and with a few tweaks, it can be made healthier. Start by making a simple sponge cake using almond flour, coconut oil, eggs, and honey. Top the cake with a dollop of whipped cream (made with coconut cream and honey) and fresh strawberries. For an extra kick of flavor, add a sprinkle of cinnamon to the whipped cream.

Fruit and Yogurt Parfait

This dessert is as delicious as it is beautiful. Simply layer fresh fruit (such as berries, kiwi, and mango) with Greek yogurt in a glass or parfait dish. Top with a drizzle of honey and a sprinkle of granola or chopped nuts for crunch. This dessert is not only tasty but also packed with protein and fiber.

Baked Apples

Baked apples are a comforting and healthy dessert option that's perfect for fall. To make this dessert, core and slice apples (any variety will do) and place them in a baking dish. Drizzle with maple syrup and sprinkle with cinnamon and nutmeg. Bake in the oven until the apples are tender and caramelized. Serve with a dollop of Greek yogurt or a scoop of vanilla ice cream (if desired).

Chocolate Chia Seed Pudding

Chia seeds are packed with fiber and omega-3 fatty acids, making them a superfood in their own right. Combine chia seeds with almond milk, cocoa powder, and honey for a healthy and delicious chocolate pudding. Let the pudding chill in the refrigerator for at least two hours before serving. Top with fresh berries or sliced bananas for added flavor and texture.

Frozen Banana Bites

These frozen banana bites are a fun and healthy dessert option that's perfect for kids and adults alike. Start by slicing bananas into rounds and dipping them in melted dark chocolate. Top with chopped nuts or shredded coconut (if desired) and freeze until solid. These banana bites are not only delicious but also packed with potassium and antioxidants.

Grilled Peaches with Yogurt and Honey

Grilling peaches brings out their natural sweetness and creates a deliciously caramelized flavor. Simply slice peaches in half, remove the pits, and place them cut-side down on a grill pan or outdoor grill. Grill for a few minutes on each side until the peaches are tender and caramelized. Top with Greek yogurt and a drizzle of honey for a healthy and satisfying dessert option.

Mixed Berry Sorbet

This refreshing and healthy sorbet is perfect for hot summer days. To make the sorbet, blend together mixed berries (such as strawberries, blueberries, and raspberries) with a little bit of honey and lemon juice. Freeze the mixture in an ice cream maker until it's firm. Serve the sorbet with fresh berries or a sprig of mint for an extra burst of flavor.

No-Bake Energy Balls

These no-bake energy balls are a delicious and healthy snack option that can double as a dessert. To make the energy balls, simply combine rolled oats, nut butter, honey, chia seeds, and mini chocolate chips in a bowl. Form the mixture into small balls and refrigerate until firm. These energy balls are not only tasty but also packed with protein and fiber, making them a great post-workout snack.

Sweet Potato Brownies

Yes, you read that right - sweet potato brownies! These brownies are a healthy and decadent dessert option that's perfect for chocoholics. To make the brownies, combine mashed sweet potato, almond flour, cocoa powder, honey, and eggs in a bowl. Bake the mixture in a baking dish until the brownies are set. Top with a drizzle of melted dark chocolate (if desired) and serve.

Desserts don't have to be unhealthy, and these dessert ideas and recipes prove just that. With a little creativity and the right ingredients, you can indulge in your sweet tooth without sabotaging your diet. Whether you're in the mood for chocolate pudding, grilled peaches, or energy balls, there's a healthy dessert option for everyone. So go ahead and indulge - your taste buds (and your waistline) will thank you.

Eating out can be a challenge for anyone trying to maintain a healthy diet, but it can be especially difficult for people with type 2 diabetes. With limited control over the ingredients and preparation methods, it can be challenging to make healthy choices while still enjoying the experience of dining out. However, with the right strategies in place, it is possible to manage your blood sugar levels and still enjoy eating out with friends and family. In this article, we will discuss some effective strategies for eating out with type 2 diabetes.

Plan Ahead

One of the most important strategies for eating out with type 2 diabetes is to plan ahead. This means doing some research before heading out to a restaurant. Many restaurants have their menus available online, so take some time to review the menu and identify the healthier options.

Look for dishes that are high in protein, fiber, and healthy fats, and low in refined carbohydrates and added sugars.

Another important aspect of planning ahead is to make sure you know your portion sizes. Many restaurants serve larger portions than what is recommended for a healthy diet, which can make it difficult to manage your blood sugar levels. Consider sharing a meal with a friend or taking half of your meal home for later.

Communicate with Your Server

When dining out with type 2 diabetes, it is important to communicate with your server. Let them know about your dietary restrictions and ask for modifications to your meal if necessary. For example, if a dish comes with a side of French fries, ask if you can substitute a salad or steamed vegetables instead. Most restaurants are happy to accommodate dietary restrictions, so don't be afraid to speak up.

It is also a good idea to ask your server about the preparation methods for the dishes you are interested in.

For example, if you are ordering grilled chicken, ask if it is marinated in sugar or if it is cooked with added oils or butter. This will help you make more informed decisions about what to order.

Be Mindful of Hidden Sugars

Hidden sugars can be a challenge when dining out with type 2 diabetes. Many sauces, dressings, and marinades contain added sugars, which can significantly impact your blood sugar levels. When ordering, ask for sauces and dressings on the side so you can control the amount you consume. You can also ask for lemon wedges or vinegar and oil as a healthier alternative to sugary dressings.

Another way to avoid hidden sugars is to avoid dishes that are breaded or fried. These types of dishes often contain added sugars in the breading or coating. Instead, look for grilled, baked, or broiled options.

Choose Your Beverages Wisely

Beverages can also impact your blood sugar levels when dining out with type 2 diabetes. Sugary drinks like soda, sweet tea, and lemonade can cause a rapid increase in blood sugar levels. Instead, choose water, unsweetened iced tea, or diet soda as a healthier alternative.

If you choose to have an alcoholic beverage, it is important to do so in moderation. Alcohol can cause a decrease in blood sugar levels, so be sure to monitor your levels closely. It is also important to avoid sugary mixed drinks and opt for a light beer or a glass of wine instead.

Focus on Whole Foods

When dining out with type 2 diabetes, it is important to focus on whole foods. Whole foods are foods that are minimally processed and contain no added sugars. Examples of whole foods include fresh fruits and vegetables, lean proteins, and whole grains.

One way to ensure you are getting whole foods when dining out is to choose dishes that are made with whole ingredients. For example, a salad with fresh greens, grilled chicken, and avocado is a healthier option than a salad with processed meats, croutons, and sugary dressings. Similarly, a stir-fry made with fresh vegetables, lean protein, and brown rice is a better option than a dish made with fried noodles and heavy sauces.

Consider Timing

The timing of your meals when dining out can also impact your blood sugar levels. Eating a large meal late at night can cause a spike in blood sugar levels, which can be difficult to manage. It is best to eat smaller meals throughout the day to maintain stable blood sugar levels.

When dining out, consider scheduling your meal earlier in the day or ordering smaller portions. You can also ask your server to pack up half of your meal for later, so you can enjoy the rest at a more appropriate time.

Don't Be Afraid to Ask for Help

Managing type 2 diabetes can be challenging, and it's okay to ask for help when dining out. Consider bringing a friend or family member who can help you make healthier choices and support you in managing your blood sugar levels. You can also consider working with a registered dietitian who can provide personalized recommendations and support.

Chapter 8
Managing Your Blood Sugar

Blood sugar management is crucial for people with diabetes. High blood sugar levels can lead to a range of complications, from nerve damage to cardiovascular disease. Managing blood sugar levels involves a combination of diet, exercise, and medication. In this article, we'll explore strategies for managing blood sugar levels, including lifestyle changes and medications.

Eat a Healthy Diet

The foods you eat can have a significant impact on your blood sugar levels. To manage your blood sugar levels, it's essential to eat a healthy diet that's low in carbohydrates and high in fiber. Carbohydrates are the main nutrient that raises blood sugar levels, so limiting your carbohydrate intake is a key part of managing blood sugar levels.

Some of the best foods to eat when you're managing blood sugar levels include:

- Non-starchy vegetables: Broccoli, spinach, cauliflower, and other non-starchy vegetables are low in carbohydrates and high in fiber, making them an excellent choice for people with diabetes.

- Whole grains: Whole grains, such as brown rice, quinoa, and whole-grain bread, are a good source of fiber and are less likely to cause blood sugar spikes than refined grains.

- Lean protein: Lean protein, such as chicken, turkey, fish, and tofu, can help keep you feeling full and satisfied, which can help you avoid overeating and keep your blood sugar levels stable.

- Healthy fats: Avocado, nuts, and olive oil are all good sources of healthy fats that can help improve blood sugar control.

Exercise Regularly

Exercise is another essential strategy for managing blood sugar levels. When you exercise, your muscles use glucose for energy, which can help lower your blood sugar levels. Regular exercise can also help you lose weight, which can improve blood sugar control.

The American Diabetes Association recommends that people with diabetes aim for at least 150 minutes of moderate-intensity aerobic exercise per week. Some good exercises for people with diabetes include walking, cycling, swimming, and yoga.

If you're new to exercise or have other health conditions, it's essential to talk to your doctor before starting a new exercise program. Your doctor can help you create an exercise plan that's safe and effective for you.

Monitor Your Blood Sugar Levels

Monitoring your blood sugar levels regularly is a crucial part of managing diabetes. Regular blood sugar monitoring can help you identify trends and patterns in your blood sugar levels, which can help you make adjustments to your diet, exercise, and medication as needed.

The frequency of blood sugar monitoring can vary depending on your specific needs and the recommendations of your doctor. Some people may need to check their blood sugar levels several times a day, while others may need to check their blood sugar levels less frequently.

Take Your Medications as Directed

Medication is often an essential part of managing blood sugar levels. There are several types of medications that can help lower blood sugar levels, including:

- Metformin: Metformin is a medication that can help lower blood sugar levels by reducing glucose production in the liver.
- Sulfonylureas: Sulfonylureas are a type of medication that can help stimulate insulin production in the pancreas, which can help lower blood sugar levels.
- DPP-4 inhibitors: DPP-4 inhibitors are a type of medication that can help lower blood sugar levels by increasing insulin production in response to glucose.
- Insulin: Insulin is a hormone that regulates blood sugar levels. People with type 1 diabetes need to take insulin to survive, while people with type 2

diabetes may need to take insulin to help manage their blood sugar levels.

It's essential to take your medications as directed by your doctor. Missing doses or taking medications incorrectly can lead to high or low blood sugar levels, which can be dangerous.

Manage Stress

Stress can have a significant impact on blood sugar levels. When you're stressed, your body releases hormones like cortisol and adrenaline, which can cause blood sugar levels to rise. Chronic stress can also make it more difficult to manage diabetes by making it harder to stick to a healthy diet and exercise routine.

Managing stress is essential for people with diabetes. Some strategies for managing stress include:

- Exercise: Exercise is a great way to reduce stress and improve blood sugar control at the same time.

- Mindfulness meditation: Mindfulness meditation can help reduce stress by increasing awareness and acceptance of the present moment.

- Yoga: Yoga combines physical exercise with mindfulness meditation, making it an excellent way to reduce stress and improve blood sugar control.

- Relaxation techniques: Techniques like deep breathing, progressive muscle relaxation, and guided imagery can help reduce stress and improve blood sugar control.

Get Enough Sleep

Getting enough sleep is crucial for people with diabetes. Sleep deprivation can cause blood sugar levels to rise, and it can also make it more challenging to manage diabetes by making it harder to stick to a healthy diet and exercise routine.

The National Sleep Foundation recommends that adults aim for seven to nine hours of sleep per night. Some tips for getting better sleep include:

- Stick to a consistent sleep schedule: Try to go to bed and wake up at the same time every day, even on weekends.

- Create a relaxing bedtime routine: Develop a routine that helps you wind down and relax before bed.

- Make your bedroom conducive to sleep: Keep your bedroom cool, dark, and quiet.

- Limit caffeine and alcohol: Caffeine and alcohol can interfere with sleep, so it's best to avoid them in the hours leading up to bedtime.

CONCLUSION

A healthier lifestyle is essential for managing type 2 diabetes. Research has shown that a healthy diet, regular exercise, and weight loss can improve blood sugar control and reduce the risk of complications associated with the condition. In addition to these physical benefits, a healthier lifestyle can also improve mental health and overall well-being.

Dietary Changes

One of the most significant lifestyle changes that individuals with type 2 diabetes can make is to adopt a healthier diet. A healthy diet should be rich in whole foods, such as fruits, vegetables, whole grains, lean protein, and healthy fats. These foods provide essential nutrients and can help improve blood sugar control.

To start making dietary changes, it is essential to understand what types of foods to eat and what to avoid. For example, individuals with type 2 diabetes should limit their intake of refined carbohydrates, such as white bread and sugary drinks, which can cause blood sugar spikes. Instead, they should focus on eating foods that are low in carbohydrates, such as non-starchy vegetables and lean protein sources.

Regular Exercise

Regular exercise is also essential for managing type 2 diabetes. Exercise helps improve blood sugar control by increasing insulin sensitivity and reducing insulin resistance. It also helps individuals maintain a healthy weight and reduces the risk of developing cardiovascular disease, which is a common complication of diabetes.

Getting started with exercise can be challenging, especially if an individual has not exercised regularly in the past. However, it is important to start slow and gradually increase the intensity and duration of exercise. Aim for at least 30 minutes of moderate-intensity exercise, such as brisk walking, most days of the week.

Weight Loss

For individuals who are overweight or obese, weight loss is an essential part of managing type 2 diabetes. Losing weight can improve blood sugar control and reduce the risk of complications associated with the condition. Even small amounts of weight loss, such as 5-10% of total body weight, can have a significant impact on blood sugar control.

To achieve weight loss, individuals should focus on creating a calorie deficit by consuming fewer calories than they burn through exercise and daily activities. This can be achieved through a combination of dietary changes and regular exercise.

Tips for Starting a Healthier Lifestyle with Type 2 Diabetes

Starting a healthier lifestyle with type 2 diabetes can be challenging, but there are many tips and strategies that can help individuals get started.

1. Set Realistic Goals: When starting a healthier lifestyle, it is important to set realistic goals. This means setting goals that are achievable and sustainable. For example, instead of setting a goal to lose 50 pounds in three months, set a goal to lose 1-2 pounds per week over the next six months. This is a more achievable goal and is more likely to lead to long-term success.

2. Make Gradual Changes: Making too many changes at once can be overwhelming and lead to failure. Instead, start by making small, gradual changes to your diet and exercise routine. For example, start by adding a daily walk or replacing sugary drinks with water.

3. Stay Motivated: Staying motivated can be challenging when making lifestyle changes, especially when progress is slow. To stay motivated, set small goals and celebrate when you achieve them. You can also track your progress and use a journal or app to monitor your daily activities and progress.

4. Focus on the Benefits: When starting a healthier lifestyle, it can be easy to focus on the challenges and difficulties of making changes. Instead, focus on the benefits of a healthier lifestyle. For example, remind yourself of the improved blood sugar control, increased energy, and reduced risk of complications that come with a healthier lifestyle.